About the NCCN Guidelines for Patients®

National Comprehensive Cancer Network®

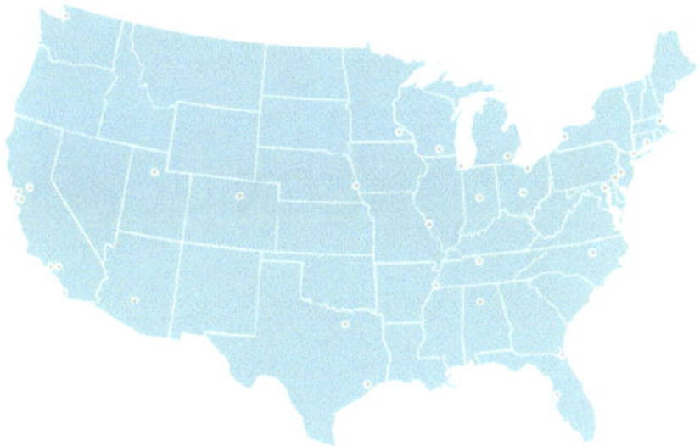

Did you know that top cancer centers across the United States work together to improve cancer care? This alliance of leading cancer centers is called the National Comprehensive Cancer Network® (NCCN®).

Cancer care is always changing. NCCN develops evidence-based cancer care recommendations used by health care providers worldwide. These frequently updated recommendations are the NCCN Clinical Practice Guidelines in Oncology (NCCN Guidelines®). The NCCN Guidelines for Patients plainly explain these expert recommendations for people with cancer and caregivers.

These NCCN Guidelines for Patients are based on the NCCN Clinical Practice Guidelines in Oncology (NCCN Guidelines®) for Neuroendocrine and Adrenal Tumors Version 2.2025 – May 28, 2025.

Learn how the NCCN Guidelines for Patients are developed
NCCN.org/patient-guidelines-process

View the NCCN Guidelines for Patients free online
NCCN.org/patientguidelines

Find an NCCN Cancer Center near you
NCCN.org/cancercenters

Connect with us

Supporters

NATIONAL COMPREHENSIVE CANCER NETWORK®
NCCN FOUNDATION
Guiding Treatment. Changing Lives.

NCCN Guidelines for Patients are supported by funding from the NCCN Foundation®

NCCN Foundation gratefully acknowledges the following corporate supporter for helping to make available these NCCN Guidelines for Patients: Novartis Pharmaceuticals Corporation.

NCCN independently adapts, updates, and hosts the NCCN Guidelines for Patients. Our corporate supporters do not participate in the development of the NCCN Guidelines for Patients and are not responsible for the content and recommendations contained therein.

To make a gift or learn more, visit online or email

NCCNFoundation.org/Donate

PatientGuidelines@NCCN.org

Contents

NCCN Foundation seeks to support the millions of patients and their families affected by a cancer diagnosis by funding and distributing NCCN Guidelines for Patients. NCCN Foundation is also committed to advancing cancer treatment by funding the nation's promising doctors at the center of innovation in cancer research. For more details and the full library of patient and caregiver resources, visit NCCN.org/patients.

National Comprehensive Cancer Network (NCCN) and NCCN Foundation
3025 Chemical Road, Suite 100, Plymouth Meeting, PA 19462 USA

1 About adrenal tumors

The adrenal glands sit on top of the kidneys and produce hormones used throughout the body. Adrenal tumors can form in one or both adrenal glands. Most adrenal tumors are benign (not cancer) and don't cause symptoms. This chapter reviews the basics of adrenal tumors.

What's an adrenal tumor?

A tumor is a group of abnormal cells. Adrenal tumors start in the adrenal glands. Your body has 2 adrenal glands, one on top of each kidney. Adrenal glands are small, yellow organs that are important to the body's endocrine system. The endocrine system is made up of tissues and organs that produce hormones. Hormones are chemical substances that are made by the body to help control how organs or cells work.

Each adrenal gland has an inner and outer part:

- **Adrenal cortex** – This is the outer part of the adrenal gland. The adrenal cortex makes 3 main hormones: cortisol, aldosterone, and dehydroepiandrosterone (DHEA). These hormones control metabolism, blood pressure, and body features (such as hair growth and body shape).

Adrenal glands

Adrenal glands are small, triangle-shaped glands found on the top of the kidneys. These glands make hormones that help to regulate your immune system, response to stress, metabolism, and other functions.

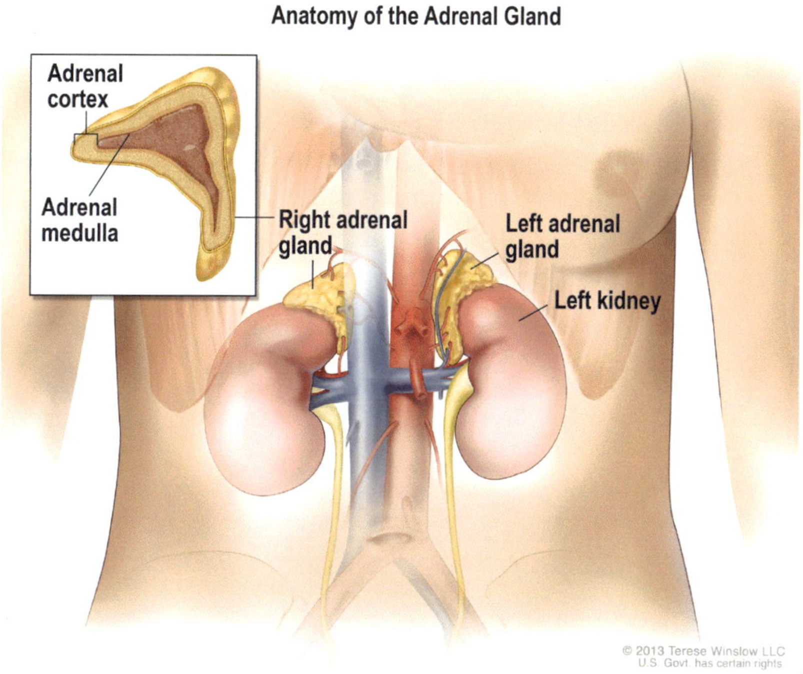

- **Adrenal medulla** – This is the inner part of the adrenal gland. The medulla makes 3 hormones: epinephrine, norepinephrine, and dopamine. These hormones control the body's response to stress.

What are the types of adrenal tumors?

Adrenal tumors are grouped in the following ways:

- **Benign (not cancer) or malignant (cancer)** – Most adrenal tumors are benign. Benign tumors don't metastasize (spread) to other parts of the body. But they can grow quickly and press on nearby organs. Certain genetic conditions may increase the risk for malignant tumors.
- **Functioning or nonfunctioning** – Functioning tumors produce excess hormones, which can sometimes cause symptoms. Symptoms depend on the type of hormone released by the tumor. Functioning tumors are usually benign, although some can become cancerous and spread. Nonfunctioning tumors don't produce extra hormones.

Adrenal tumors are also broken down into 4 types:

- **Adenoma** – This is the most common type of adrenal gland tumor, also referred to as adrenocortical adenoma. It's a benign tumor that can be functioning (produce excess hormones) or nonfunctioning.
- **Adrenocortical carcinoma (ACC)** – An ACC is a type of cancer that begins in the adrenal cortex (outer layer) of the adrenal gland. It can be a functioning or nonfunctioning tumor. If the tumor is functioning, it may produce more than 1 hormone.
- **Neuroblastoma** – This type of adrenal tumor is cancerous. It affects children ages 5 and under, though it is most often found in infants. Neuroblastoma can spread to other parts of the body, including the bones.
- **Pheochromocytoma (PCC)** – This type of tumor begins in the adrenal medulla (inner part) of the adrenal gland. It can cause high blood pressure, headaches, rapid heartbeat, and sweating. Most PCCs are benign, but occasionally can be cancerous.

The term adrenal tumor will be used throughout this guide to mean adrenal tumors in general and not a specific type.

How are adrenal tumors diagnosed and treated?

Most adrenal tumors are found through imaging tests done for an unrelated issue. Many of these tumors can just be observed, but some will require surgery to remove the tumor with the whole adrenal gland.

This guide will discuss in greater detail how adrenal tumors are diagnosed and treated. It'll provide an overview of the types of tests and treatments and what to expect during testing and treatment.

How can I get the best care?

Advocate for yourself. You have an important role to play in your care. Many people feel more satisfied when they actively take part in planning their cancer care.

The NCCN Guidelines for Patients will help you play a larger role in your care. Discuss the recommendations in this guide with your care team. Ask questions about your options and share your goals and concerns.

Don’t know what to ask? You’re not alone. That’s why we include suggested questions to ask at the end of chapter.

Keep reading to find the best care for you.

How this guide can help you

Making decisions about cancer care is stressful. There’s a lot to learn, and you don’t know what the future holds.

Use this guide to get the information and support you need.

Patients, doctors, and other health care professionals trust the NCCN Guidelines for Patients. This guide uses clear, everyday language to explain current cancer care recommendations made by respected experts in the field. Their recommendations are based on the latest research and practices at leading cancer centers.

Your health is unique to you, so your cancer care should be, too. As you read this guide, you’ll learn which treatments are likely to provide the best results for you. And you’ll be better prepared to talk with your care team.

2

Testing for adrenal tumors

Treatment planning starts with testing. Your care team will want to gather as much information as they can about your adrenal tumor. This chapter presents an overview of the possible tests you might receive and what to expect.

Tests are used to find tumors, plan treatment, and see how your tumor is responding to treatment. Results from blood and urine tests, and imaging studies will be used to determine what treatments are best for your type of adrenal tumor. This chapter provides a general overview of some of the tests you might have.

General health tests

Some general health tests are described next.

Medical history

A medical or health history is a record of all health issues and treatments you have had in your life. It asks about past surgeries and current health conditions. Bring a list of old and new medicines and any over-the-counter medicines, herbals, or supplements you take. Some supplements interact with and affect medicines that your care team may prescribe. Also, tell your care team about any symptoms you have.

Family history

Some tumors, cancers, and other diseases can run in families. Your doctor will ask about the health history of family members who are blood relatives. This information is called a

"Be your own advocate. Talk to someone who has gone through the same thing as you. Ask a lot of questions, even the ones you are afraid to ask. You have to protect yourself and ensure you make the best decisions for you, and get the best care for your particular situation."

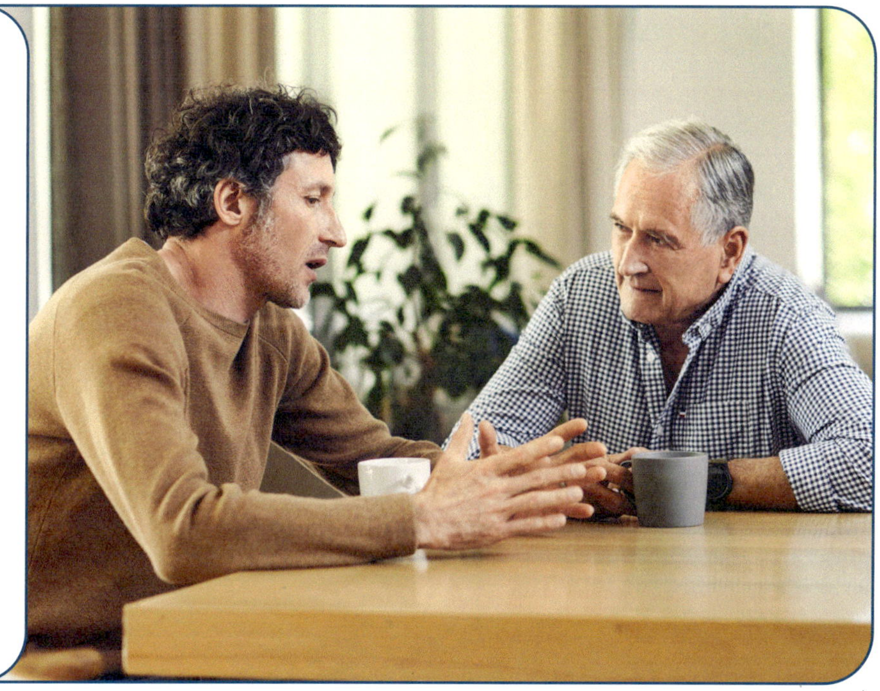

family history. Ask family members on both sides of your family about their health issues like heart disease, cancer, and diabetes, and at what age they were diagnosed. It's important to know the specific type of cancer, where the cancer started, if it's in multiple locations, and if they had genetic testing.

Physical exam

During a physical exam, your health care team may:

- Check your temperature, blood pressure, pulse, and breathing rate
- Check your height and weight
- Listen to your lungs and heart
- Look in your eyes, ears, nose, and throat
- Feel and apply pressure to parts of your body to see if organs are of normal size, are soft or hard, or cause pain when touched.
- Feel for enlarged lymph nodes in your neck, underarm, and groin.

Performance status

Performance status is a rating of a person's general level of fitness and ability to perform daily tasks. It's one factor taken into consideration when choosing a treatment plan.

Blood and urine tests

Blood and urine tests check for signs of disease and how well organs are working. They are also used to look for hormones and other chemicals produced by your tumor. Blood tests require a sample of blood, which is removed through a needle placed into a vein in your arm. For a urine test, you'll be asked to fill a small container with urine (pee in a cup). Blood and urine samples are sent to a lab for testing.

Some possible blood and urine tests are described next.

Biochemical tests

There are many types of biochemical tests. They measure substances such as hormones, proteins, and sugar (glucose) in blood and urine. You might be asked to fast (not eat) or to collect your urine at home for 24 hours using a special container.

Complete blood count

A complete blood count (CBC) measures the levels of red blood cells, white blood cells, and platelets in your blood. A CBC is a key test that gives a picture of your overall health.

Comprehensive metabolic panel

A comprehensive metabolic panel measures substances in your blood. It provides important information about how well your kidneys and liver are working, among other things.

Adrenal vein sampling

Adrenal vein sampling measures how much of the hormone aldosterone is produced by each adrenal gland. This procedure is done by inserting a needle and catheter (plastic tube) into the adrenal veins and taking blood coming directly from each adrenal gland. Adrenal vein sampling is used to diagnose primary aldosteronism (Conn syndrome), a condition that causes the adrenal glands to produce too much aldosterone.

Imaging tests

You'll likely have a combination of imaging tests. Imaging tests take pictures of the inside of your body. They show the primary tumor, or where the cancer started, and look for cancer or tumors in other parts of the body. A radiologist, a doctor who's an expert at interpreting imaging tests, will send a report to your care team. The following information isn't in order of importance.

Contrast material

Contrast material is a substance used to improve the quality of imaging tests such as CT and MRI scans. It is used to make the pictures clearer. Not all imaging tests require contrast, but many do.

Contrast might be taken by mouth (oral) or given through a vein (intravenously or IV). Oral contrast will be passed with your next bowel movements. IV contrast will leave the body in the urine immediately after the test. The types of contrast vary and are different for CT and MRI.

Tell your care team if you've had allergic reactions to contrast in the past. This is important. You might be given medicines to avoid the effects of those allergies. Contrast

CT machine

A CT machine is large and has a tunnel in the middle. During the test, you will lie on the table, which moves slowly through the tunnel.

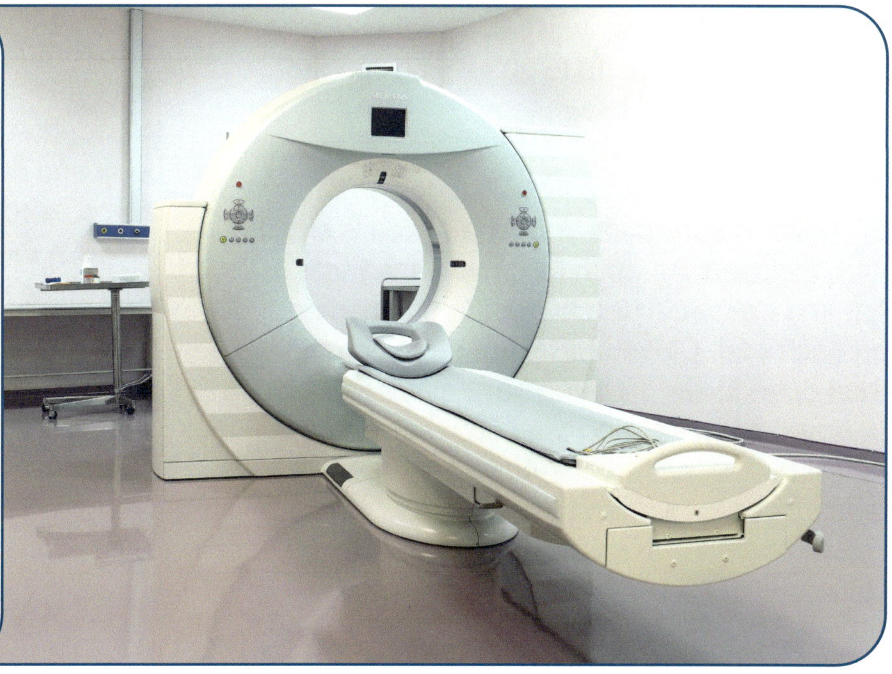

might not be used if you have a serious allergy or if your kidneys aren't working well.

CT scan

A computed tomography (CT or CAT) scan uses x-rays and computer technology to take pictures of the inside of the body. It takes many x-rays of the same body part from different angles.

Other less common types of CT scans such as a single-photon emission computed tomography (SPECT) and 4D-CT may be used in very specific cases.

MRI scan

A magnetic resonance imaging (MRI) scan uses radio waves and powerful magnets to take pictures of the inside of the body. It doesn't use x-rays, which means there's no radiation delivered to your body during the test. Because of the very strong magnets used in the MRI machine, tell the technologist if you have any metal or a pacemaker in your body. During the test, you'll likely be asked to hold your breath for 10 to 20 seconds as the technician collects the images.

A closed MRI has a capsule-like design where the magnet surrounds you. The space is small and enclosed. An open MRI has a magnetic top and bottom, which allows for an opening on each end. Closed MRIs are more common than open MRIs, so if you have claustrophobia (a dread or fear of enclosed spaces), be sure to talk to your care team about it. MRI scans take longer to perform than CT scans.

Multiphasic CT or MRI

In a multiphasic CT or MRI there are 2 scans, one without contrast and one with contrast. First, a scan is done without contrast. Then, contrast is injected into a vein and multiple sets of pictures are taken as the contrast moves through the area of the body near the tumor. This allows your care team to see whether the tumor involves any veins, arteries, or organs.

MIBG scan

An MIBG scan uses a radiotracer called iodine meta-iodobenzylguanidine (MIBG). A special camera detects the tracer and takes pictures of the inside of your body. An (MIBG) scan is done in stages over several days and is different than a PET scan. An MIBG scan might be done with single-photon emission CT called a SPECT/CT to enhance the quality of the images.

PET scan

A PET (positron emission tomography) scan uses a radioactive substance called a tracer that's injected into a vein. On the scan, the tracer shows where cancer cells are in the body and how much sugar is being taken up by the cancer cells. This gives an idea about how fast the cancer cells are growing. Cancer cells show up as bright spots on PET scans. However, not all tumors will appear on a PET scan. Also, not all bright spots found on the PET scan are cancer. It's normal for the brain, heart, kidneys, and bladder to be bright on a PET scan. Inflammation or infection can also show up as a bright spot.

A PET scan can be combined with a CT, MRI, or SSTR.

The following are types of PET scans that might be used for adrenal tumors:

- **FDG-PET** uses a radiotracer called fluorodeoxyglucose (FDG) that's made of fluoride and a simple form of sugar called glucose. FDG-PET scans can help determine if tumors are becoming more aggressive or when there is cancer in the bones. An FDG-PET might be combined with an SSTR-PET to provide more detailed information about the tumor.
- **SSTR-PET** uses a tracer that binds to somatostatin receptors (SSTRs). Somatostatin is a hormone that helps to control other hormones in the body.
- **SSTR-PET/CT or SSTR-PET/MRI** adds CT or MRI to an SSTR-PET to help improve accuracy and find out if tumor cells have SSTRs.

Biopsy

A biopsy is the removal of a sample of tissue or group of cells for testing. It's an important part of an accurate diagnosis. A pathologist, a doctor who identifies diseases by studying cells and tissues, will examine the biopsy sample and note the overall appearance and the size, shape, and type of cells. This is called histology or histopathology. **Biopsies are rarely done on adrenal tumors.** Instead, lab tests are done on the tumor after it's removed.

Some types of biopsies may include:

- **Fine-needle aspiration or core biopsy** uses needles of different sizes to remove a sample of tissue or fluid.
- **Liquid biopsy** uses a sample of blood for testing.

Genetic testing

Depending on your family history or other features of your tumor, your health care team might refer you for hereditary genetic testing to learn more about your tumor. A genetic counselor or trained provider will speak with you about the results.

Genetic testing is done using blood or saliva (spitting into a cup or taking a cheek swab). The goal is to look for gene mutations inherited from your biological (birth) parents called germline mutations. Some genetic mutations can put you at risk for more than one type of tumor or cancer. You can pass these mutations on to your children. Also, other family members might carry these mutations. Tell your care team if there is a family history of cancer.

Hereditary cancer predisposition syndromes

Certain genetic (inherited) syndromes may put someone at risk for developing certain tumors and cancers. A syndrome is a group of signs or symptoms that occur together and suggest the presence of or risk for a disease. A hereditary syndrome may also be found in blood (biological) relatives.

A genetic cancer risk assessment will identify if you have a genetic risk factor for tumors or cancer, if you may benefit from genetic testing, additional screening, or preventive interventions. Depending on the genetic risk assessment, you might undergo genetic testing and genetic counseling to see if you have a hereditary syndrome that puts you at risk for developing adrenal tumors.

For hereditary syndromes related to tumors found in or near the adrenal glands, **see Guide 1.**

Biomarker testing

A sample from a biopsy of your tumor may be tested to look for gene mutations, protein levels, or other molecular features. It's sometimes called molecular testing or tumor profiling, tumor sequencing, gene expression profiling, or genomic testing. Your treatment team will recommend the best types of biomarker testing that are important for you.

Immunohistochemistry

Immunohistochemistry (IHC) is a special staining process used to study cells from a biopsy or tumor sample. Examples of biomarkers found with IHC might include synaptophysin, chromogranin A, S-100 Immunostain, INSM1, and keratins.

Guide 1
Hereditary syndromes

Adrenocortical carcinoma (ACC)	• Li-Fraumeni syndrome, *TP53* gene affected • Lynch syndrome, genes affected include *MLH1, EPCAM/MSH2, MSH6, PMS2* • Multiple endocrine neoplasia type 1 (MEN1), *MEN1* gene affected • Familial adenomatous polyposis (APC)
Adrenal adenoma	• MEN1
Pheochromocytoma (PCC)	• Hereditary PCC/PGL syndrome, genes affected include *MAX, SDHA, SDHAF2, SDHB, SDHC, SDHD,* or *TMEM127* • Multiple endocrine neoplasia type 2 (MEN2), *RET* gene affected • Neurofibromatosis type 1, *NF1* gene affected • Von Hippel-Lindau (VHL) syndrome
Paraganglioma (PGL)	• Hereditary PCC/PGL syndrome • VHL syndrome

Key points

- Tests are used to find tumors, plan treatment, and check how your tumor or cancer is responding to treatment.
- Results from blood and urine tests, and imaging studies will be used to determine what treatments are best for your type of tumor.
- Blood and urine tests look for signs of disease and how well your organs are working. These tests are also used to measure hormone, blood sugar (glucose), and protein levels.
- Imaging tests take pictures of the inside of your body and are used to learn more about the type, size, and location of your tumor.
- A biopsy is the removal of a sample of tissue or group of cells for testing. Biopsies are rarely done for adrenal tumors. Instead, lab tests are done on the tumor after it's removed.
- Genetic testing looks for gene mutations inherited from your biological (birth) parents called germline mutations.
- Some genetic (hereditary) conditions can put you at risk for developing an adrenal tumor. Genetic testing is often offered to people with adrenal tumors or cancer.

Questions to ask

- What tests will I have?
- What tests will be done on the tumor?
- Who will explain the test results to me?
- What other information do you need to gather before I start treatment?
- Do you recommend I have genetic testing and counseling for inherited cancer risk or predisposition syndromes? Why or why not?

3
Types of treatment

There's more than one treatment for adrenal tumors. This chapter describes treatment options and what to expect. Together, you and your care team will choose a treatment plan that's best for you.

Results from blood, urine, tumor, and imaging tests will guide your treatment plan. Many factors play a role in how a tumor or cancer responds to treatment. It's important to have regular talks with your care team about your goals for treatment and your treatment plan.

Most adrenal tumors are benign (not cancer) and don't need any treatment. These tumors will be observed with imaging studies (usually CT scan or MRI) and blood and urine tests. However, observation is not an option for everyone. Hormone-producing (functioning) tumors and cancerous adrenal tumors do require treatment. Treatment for adrenal tumors is usually a combination of therapies starting with surgery and might include systemic (drug) therapy or radiation therapy.

Your care team

Treating cancer takes a team approach. Treatment decisions should involve a multidisciplinary team of health care and psychosocial care professionals from different professional backgrounds who have knowledge and experience in your type of cancer. This team is united in the planning and implementation of your treatment. Ask who will coordinate your care.

Some members of your care team will be with you throughout cancer treatment, while others will only be there for parts of it. Get to know your care team and help them get to know you.

Your care team

Depending on the type and location of your adrenal tumor, your care team might include the following specialists.

- **Oncologist** is a doctor who diagnoses and treats cancer. Types of oncologists include medical, radiation, and surgical oncologists.
- **Endocrinologist** is a doctor who diagnoses and treats disorders of the endocrine glands.
- **Pathologist** is a doctor who analyzes the cells, tissues, and organs removed during a biopsy or surgery.
- **Radiologist** is a doctor who interprets the results of CT scans, MRIs, and other imaging tests, and performs needle biopsies as needed.

Surgery

Surgery is an operation or procedure to remove a tumor from the body. It's the main or primary treatment for adrenal tumors. Surgery is sometimes called resection or excision. Ask your care team what will be removed during surgery and what to expect.

When preparing for surgery, seek the opinion of a surgeon who is an expert in performing your type of surgery. Hospitals that perform many surgeries often have better results. You can ask for a referral to a hospital or cancer center that has experience in treating your type of cancer.

Goal of surgery

The goal of surgery or tumor resection is to remove all the cancer. To do so, the tumor is removed along with a rim of normal-looking tissue around its edge called the surgical margin. The surgical margin may look normal during surgery, but cancerous cells may be found when viewed under a microscope by a pathologist. A clear or negative margin (R0) is when no cancer cells are found in the tissue around the edge of the tumor. In a positive margin, cancer cells are found in normal-looking tissue around the tumor.

After surgery, you may receive treatment such as radiation or systemic (drug) therapy to kill any remaining cancer cells.

The kidney and adrenal gland

An adrenal gland sits on top of each kidney. The kidney and adrenal gland are surrounded by a layer of fatty tissue. Surrounding the fat is a layer of fibrous tissue called Gerota's fascia.

Derivative work of Kidney and Adrenal Gland by Alan Hoofring from NCI Visuals Online. Available at: https://visualsonline.cancer.gov/details.cfm?imageid=4355

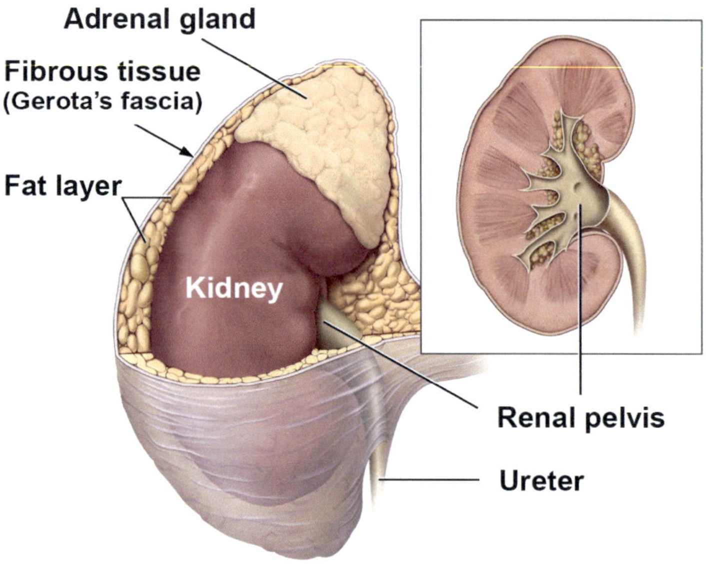

National Cancer Institute

Some examples of surgical procedures are described next. Your care team can provide more information about surgery specific to your type of tumor or cancer.

Adrenalectomy

An adrenalectomy is surgery to remove one (unilateral) or both (bilateral) adrenal glands. The tumor and any areas where the cancer has spread, including lymph nodes or nearby structures, might be removed.

There are 2 types of adrenalectomies:

- **Minimally invasive surgery** or key-hole surgery uses several small incisions. Small tools are inserted through each incision to perform the surgery. One of the tools, called a videoscope, is a long tube with a video camera at the end. The camera lets your surgeon see the area near the tumor. Other tools are used to remove the tumor. Minimally invasive surgery, also called laparoscopic surgery, can be done using robotic arms to control surgical tools. This is called robot-assisted or robotic surgery.
- **Open surgery** or laparotomy removes tissue through one large surgical cut. The large cut lets your surgeon directly view and access the tumor in your adrenal gland. Open surgery is often done when the tumor might be in lymph nodes or other nearby organs, or if cancer is suspected.

Systemic therapy

Systemic therapy is drug therapy that works throughout the body. Some types of systemic therapy include chemotherapy, targeted therapy, and immunotherapy.

All systemic treatments listed in this guide are recommended and appropriate. When helpful, NCCN experts also assign a level of preference to their recommendations for systemic therapies:

- **Preferred therapies** have the most evidence they may work better and may be safer than other therapies.
- **Other recommended therapies** can provide effective results but may have less evidence, more side effects, or may not work quite as well as preferred therapies.
- **Therapies used in certain cases** work best for individuals with specific cancer features or health circumstances.

Systemic therapy options will depend on the type of tumor. For a general list of systemic therapies, **see Guide 2.**

Chemotherapy

Chemotherapy kills fast-dividing cells throughout the body, including cancer cells and some normal cells. More than one chemotherapy may be used to treat cancer. When only one drug is used, it's called a single agent. A combination or multi-agent regimen is the use of 2 or more chemotherapy drugs.

Some chemotherapy drugs are liquids given through a vein (intravenously or IV) or injected under the skin with a needle. Other chemotherapy drugs may be given as a pill that is swallowed.

Most chemotherapy is given in cycles of treatment days followed by days of rest. This allows the body to recover before the next cycle. Cycles vary in length depending on which drugs are used. The number of treatment days per cycle and the total number of cycles given also vary.

Guide 2
Systemic therapy examples

Chemotherapy	• Carboplatin • Cisplatin • Cyclophosphamide (Frindovyx) • Dacarbazine • Doxorubicin	• Etoposide (Etopophos) • Mitotane (Lysodren) • Temozolomide (Temodar) • Vincristine
Targeted therapy	• Belzutifan (Welireg) • Cabozantinib (Cabometyx) • Dabrafenib (Tafinlar) • Metyrosine (Demser)	• Selpercatinib (Retevmo) • Sunitinib (Sutent) • Trametinib (Mekinist)
Immunotherapy	• Pembrolizumab (Keytruda) • Nivolumab (Opdivo) • Ipilimumab (Yervoy)	
Radiopharmaceutical	• High-specific-activity (HSA) iobenguane I-131 or other 131I-MIBG • PRRT with lutetium Lu 177 dotatate (Lutathera)	
Somatostatin analogs	• Octreotide LAR (Sandostatin LAR Depot) • Lanreotide (Somatuline Depot) • Octreotide acetate (Sandostatin, Bynfezia Pen)	

Targeted therapy

Targeted therapy is drug therapy that focuses on specific or unique features of cancer cells. Targeted therapies seek out how cancer cells grow, divide, and move in the body. These drugs stop or block the action of molecules that help cancer cells grow and/or survive. Some target a specific tumor (gene) mutation, such as *NTRK*. There are a few types of targeted therapies that may be used to treat adrenal tumors such as tyrosine kinase inhibitors (TKIs) and those explained next.

Somatostatin analogs

Somatostatin analogs (SSAs) and somatostatin receptor (SSTR) therapy are used to slow down or stop tumor hormone production. This helps reduce symptoms such as diarrhea and flushing and to control tumor growth. SSAs work for a long time in the body. Treatment focused on somatostatin receptors could include SSAs, PRRT, or other drugs that bind to SSTRs.

Octreotide LAR or lanreotide might be used if the tumor is SSTR-positive and/or you're having hormone-related symptoms. Octreotide acetate might be added to octreotide LAR or lanreotide.

PRRT

Peptide receptor radionuclide therapy (PRRT) combines a protein that binds to the tumor cell receptors with a radioactive element called a radionuclide. PRRT with lutetium Lu 177 dotatate may be used to slow down or stop tumor growth in SSTR-positive tumors. The treatment works by attaching to somatostatin receptors found on the tumor. This allows a high dose of radiation to be delivered directly to the tumor. Typically, this involves a series of

Standard of care is the best-known way to treat a particular disease based on past clinical trials. There may be more than one treatment that's considered standard of care. Ask your care team what treatment options are available and if a clinical trial might be right for you.

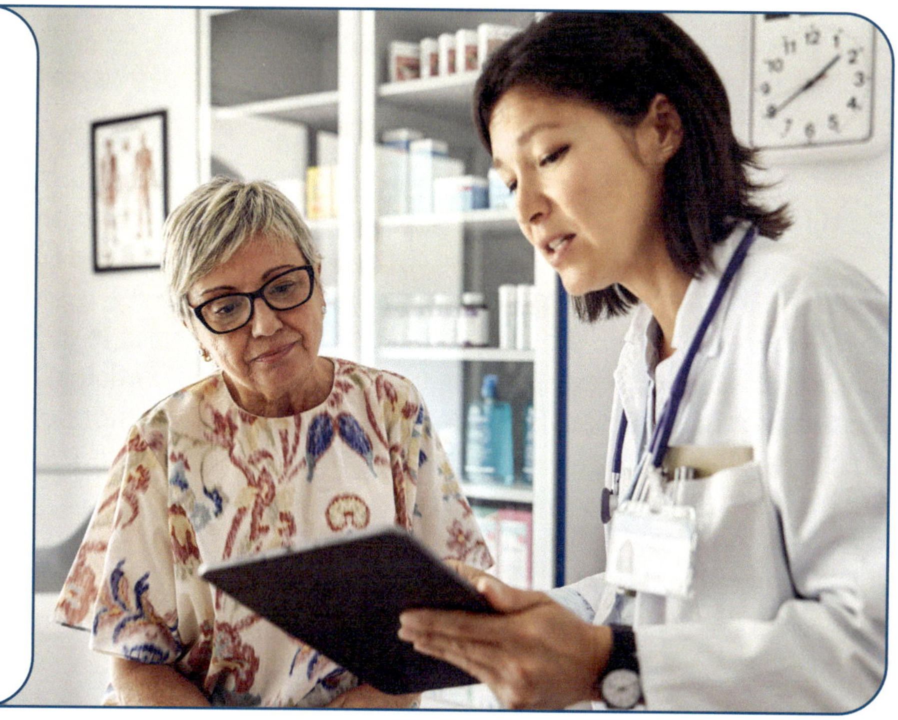

4 treatments given 8 weeks apart. PRRT is a type of radiopharmaceutical.

Radiopharmaceuticals

A radiopharmaceutical drug contains a radioactive substance that emits radiation.

Examples include:

- High-specific-activity (HSA) iobenguane I-131 or other 131I-MIBG
- PRRT with lutetium Lu 177 dotatate

Immunotherapy

The immune system has many on and off switches. Tumors take advantage of off switches. Immunotherapy can block these off switches, which helps turn the immune system back on. Immunotherapy can be given alone or with other types of treatment. Examples of immunotherapy that might be used to treat adrenal tumors include pembrolizumab, nivolumab, and ipilimumab.

Radiation therapy

Radiation therapy uses high-energy radiation from x-rays (photons), protons, and other sources to kill cancer cells, shrink tumors, or treat liver metastases. Radiation is typically delivered from outside the body by a computerized device, which can shape the treatment to closely fit the location and size of the tumor. Treatment is given in small daily doses on weekdays, with weekends off.

At least once a week, you will meet with your radiation oncologist to review treatment results and to check for side effects, such as sunburn-like rash. Ask your care team which radiation option(s) are best for your situation.

Other therapies

Tumors found in the liver or lung may be treated with surgery or one or more of the following therapies.

Ablation

Ablation uses extreme cold, extreme heat, radio waves, microwaves, or chemicals to destroy cancer cells. It can destroy small tumors and metastases with little harm to nearby tissue. Ablation might be used if you aren't healthy enough for surgery. Tumors in the liver or lung might be treated with ablation. It might take multiple treatments to destroy the tumor or metastasis.

Arterially directed therapy

Arterially directed therapy or embolization treats tumors by injecting particles, chemotherapy, or radioactive beads directly into the blood vessels that supply the tumor(s). First, a small catheter is inserted into the artery and is guided to the tumor. Once in place, the particles, chemotherapy, or beads are injected. Tumors or metastases in the liver might be treated with arterially directed therapy.

Clinical trials

You may also be able to obtain treatment through a clinical trial. A clinical trial is a type of medical research study. After being developed and tested in a lab, potential new ways of treating cancer need to be studied in people. If found to be safe and effective in a clinical trial, a drug, device, or treatment approach may be approved by the U.S. Food and Drug Administration (FDA).

Everyone with cancer should carefully consider all of the treatment options available for their cancer type, including standard treatments and clinical trials. Talk to your doctor about whether a clinical trial may make sense for you.

Phases

Most cancer clinical trials focus on treatment and are done in phases.

- **Phase 1** trials study the safety and side effects of an investigational drug or treatment approach.
- **Phase 2** trials study how well the drug or approach works against a specific type of cancer.
- **Phase 3** trials test the drug or approach against a standard treatment. If the results are good, it may be approved by the FDA.
- **Phase 4** trials study the safety and benefit of an FDA-approved treatment.

Who can enroll?

It depends on the clinical trial's rules, called eligibility criteria. The rules may be about age, cancer type and stage, treatment history, or general health. They ensure that participants are alike in specific ways and that the trial is as safe as possible for the participants.

Informed consent

Clinical trials are managed by a research team. This group of experts will review the study with you in detail, including its purpose and the risks and benefits of joining. All of this information is also provided in an informed consent form. Read the form carefully and ask questions before signing it. Take time to discuss it with people you trust. Keep in mind that you can leave and seek treatment outside of the clinical trial at any time.

Will I get a placebo?

Placebos (inactive versions of real medicines) are almost never used alone in cancer clinical trials. It is common to receive either a placebo with a standard treatment, or a new drug with a standard treatment. You will be informed, verbally and in writing, if a placebo is part of a clinical trial before you enroll.

Are clinical trials free?

There's no fee to enroll in a clinical trial. The study sponsor pays for research-related costs, including the study drug. But you may need to pay for other services, like transportation or childcare, due to extra appointments. During the trial, you will continue to receive standard cancer care. This care is often covered by insurance.

Supportive care

Supportive care is an important part of cancer care. The goal is to improve your quality of life during and after cancer treatment. Supportive care is for everyone with cancer and their families, not just for those at the end of life. It's also known as palliative care.

Supportive care includes a wide range of services. Supportive care prevents or manages the symptoms of cancer and the side effects of cancer treatment, like pain and cancer-related fatigue. It also addresses the mental, social, emotional, and spiritual concerns faced by people with cancer.

Supportive care provides help with additional needs, such as:

- Making treatment decisions
- Coordinating your care
- Paying for care
- Planning for advanced care and end of life

Read more about the types of support you may receive in *NCCN Guidelines for Patients: Palliative Care*, available at NCCN.org/patientguidelines and on the NCCN Patient Guides for Cancer app. Palliative care is appropriate for anyone, regardless of age, cancer stage, or the need for other therapies. It focuses on physical, emotional, social, and spiritual needs that affect quality of life.

It's important to tell your care team about all of your side effects, including new or worsening symptoms.

Side effects

Cancer treatment can cause unwanted health issues called side effects. Side effects depend on many factors. These factors include the drug type and dose, length of treatment, and the person. Some side effects may just be unpleasant. Others may be harmful to one's health. Treatment can cause several side effects. Some are very serious. Tell your care team about any new or worsening symptoms.

Some possible side effects of treatment are described next.

Diarrhea or constipation

Diarrhea is frequent and watery bowel movements. Your care team will tell you how to manage diarrhea. It is important to drink lots of fluids. Constipation is also common, especially if taking certain pain medicines. Drinking fluids, staying active, and taking medicines for constipation are often recommended.

Distress

Depression, anxiety, and sleeping issues are common and are a normal part of cancer diagnosis. Talk to your care team and those with whom you feel most comfortable about how you are feeling. There are services, people, and medicine that can help relieve your distress.

Fatigue

Fatigue is extreme tiredness and inability to function due to lack of energy. Fatigue may be caused by cancer or it may be a side effect of treatment. Let your care team know how you're feeling and if fatigue is getting in the way of doing the things you enjoy. Eating a balanced diet, exercise, yoga, acupuncture, and massage therapy can help. You might be referred to a nutritionist or dietitian to help with fatigue.

Survivorship

A person is a cancer survivor from the time of diagnosis until the end of life. After treatment, your health will be monitored for side effects and the return of cancer. This is part of your survivorship care plan. It's important to keep any follow-up care and imaging test appointments. Seek routine medical care, including regular doctor visits for preventive care and cancer screening.

A personalized survivorship care plan will contain a summary of possible long-term effects of treatment called late effects, and a list of follow-up tests. Find out how your primary care provider will coordinate with specialists for your follow-up care.

Supportive care resources

More information on supportive care is available at NCCN.org/patientguidelines and on the NCCN Patient Guides for Cancer app.

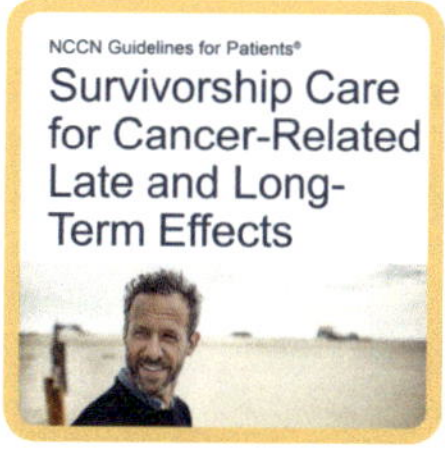

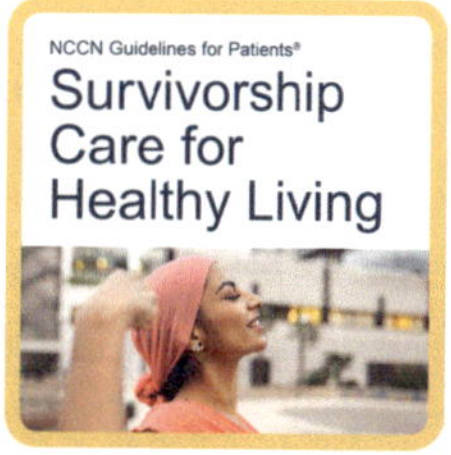

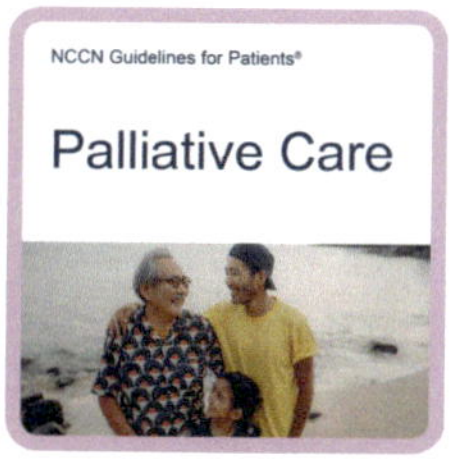

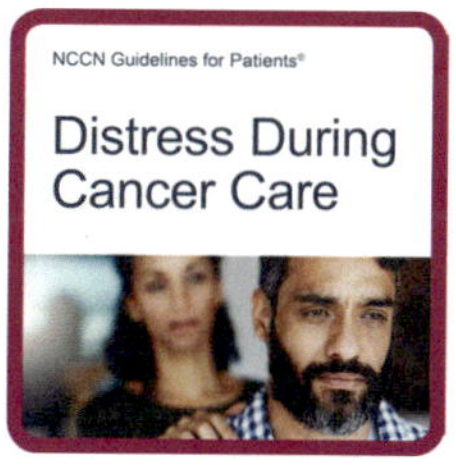

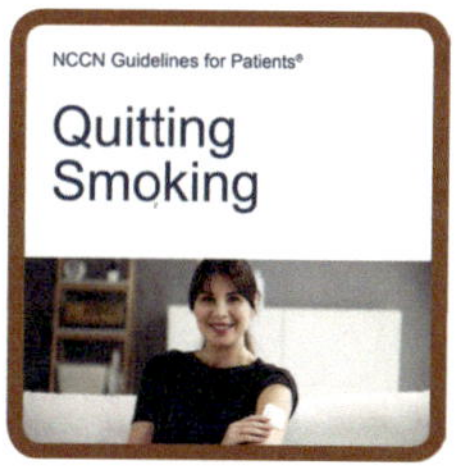

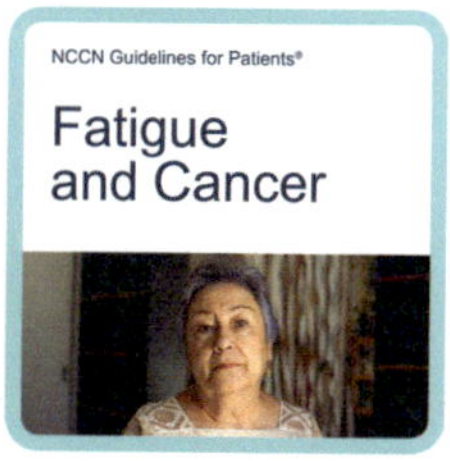

Key points

- Surgery is the main or primary treatment for adrenal tumors with limited or no spread. The type of surgery depends on where the tumor is located, the size of the tumor, and how far the disease has spread.
- Systemic therapy is drug treatment that works throughout the body. Types include chemotherapy, targeted therapy, immunotherapy, and others.
- Radiation therapy uses high-energy radiation from x-rays (photons, electrons), protons, and other sources to kill cancer cells.
- Somatostatin analogs (SSAs) and somatostatin receptor (SSTR) therapy are used to slow down or stop tumor hormone production.
- Peptide receptor radionuclide therapy (PRRT) uses a radioactive molecule to deliver high doses of radiation to destroy tumors.
- A clinical trial is a type of research that studies a treatment to see how safe it is and how well it works.
- Supportive care is health care that relieves symptoms and improves quality of life. It might include pain relief (palliative care), emotional or spiritual support, financial aid, or family counseling.

Questions to ask

- What are my treatment options?
- What treatment(s) do you recommend and why?
- What are the treatment side effects?
- Does the order of treatments matter?
- How long will treatment take?

4 Primary aldosteronism

Primary aldosteronism is a condition caused by the adrenal glands producing too much of the hormone aldosterone. Without treatment, this condition increases your risk of cardiovascular diseases, including heart attack and stroke. This chapter provides information on the testing and treatment of primary aldosteronism, also known as hyperaldosteronism or Conn syndrome.

Overview

Primary aldosteronism is a condition that occurs when one or both adrenal glands make too much aldosterone. Aldosterone is the hormone that helps to balance potassium and sodium in the body. Too much aldosterone will cause the body to hold sodium and lose potassium (hypokalemia), leading to high blood pressure (hypertension). Without treatment, this condition increases your risk of cardiovascular diseases, including heart attack and stroke. Also, low potassium levels can cause heart rhythm changes.

Primary aldosteronism is also called hyperaldosteronism or Conn syndrome.

Testing

Treatment for primary aldosteronism depends on if excess aldosterone is being produced by one or both adrenal glands. This is usually determined by a test called adrenal vein sampling, which can measure hormone levels from each adrenal gland.

Treatment

Treatment is based on whether one or both adrenal glands are producing too much aldosterone.

- **If both (bilateral) adrenal glands** are making too much aldosterone, you'll likely be treated with medicine such as spironolactone (Aldactone) or eplerenone (Inspra) to lower your blood pressure and increase potassium levels.
- **If only one (unilateral) adrenal gland** is making too much aldosterone, a minimally invasive surgery to remove the adrenal gland (adrenalectomy) is preferred. No further treatment is needed after the adrenal gland is removed.

Key points

- Primary aldosteronism occurs when one or both adrenal glands make too much aldosterone.
- Aldosterone is the hormone that helps to balance potassium and sodium in the body.
- The main symptom of primary aldosteronism is high blood pressure (hypertension) and low potassium levels (hypokalemia).
- Without treatment, this primary aldosteronism increases your risk of cardiovascular diseases, including heart attack and stroke.
- Adrenal vein sampling is a test used to determine if too much aldosterone is being produced by one or both adrenal glands.
- If both adrenal glands produce too much aldosterone, you'll be treated with medicine to lower your blood pressure and raise potassium levels. If too much aldosterone is produced by just one adrenal gland, surgery to remove the adrenal gland is recommended.

Questions to ask

- What tests will I have and what can I expect?
- Will my condition be treated with medicine or surgery? Why?
- If my condition is being treated with medicine, who will monitor my condition? A nephrologist?
- Will I take this medicine for the rest of my life?
- What are the options if the medicine doesn't lower my aldosterone levels?

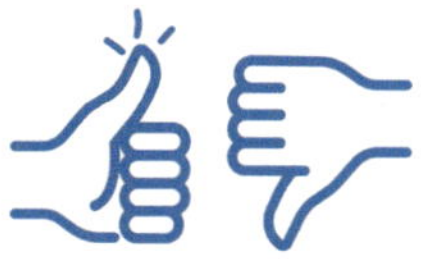

Let us know what you think!

Please take a moment to complete an online survey about the NCCN Guidelines for Patients.
NCCN.org/patients/response

5
Hypercortisolism

Cortisol is a hormone made and released by the adrenal glands. A tumor of the adrenal gland can cause too much cortisol in the body called hypercortisolism. When the body is exposed to hypercortisolism over a long period of time, a condition called Cushing syndrome can develop.

Overview

Cortisol is a hormone made and released by the adrenal glands. It helps the body use glucose (a sugar), protein, and fats. Hypercortisolemia or hypercortisolism occurs where there is too much cortisol in your body.

A tumor of the adrenal gland can cause hypercortisolism. These tumors are usually benign (not cancer). When the body is exposed to hypercortisolism over a long period of time, a condition called Cushing syndrome can develop. Without treatment, Cushing syndrome can cause facial roundness, weight gain around the middle body and upper back, thinning of the arms and legs, easy bruising, and stretch marks.

Adrenal tumors are measured in centimeters: A baseball is 7 cm, a golf ball is 4 cm, and a pea is 1 cm.

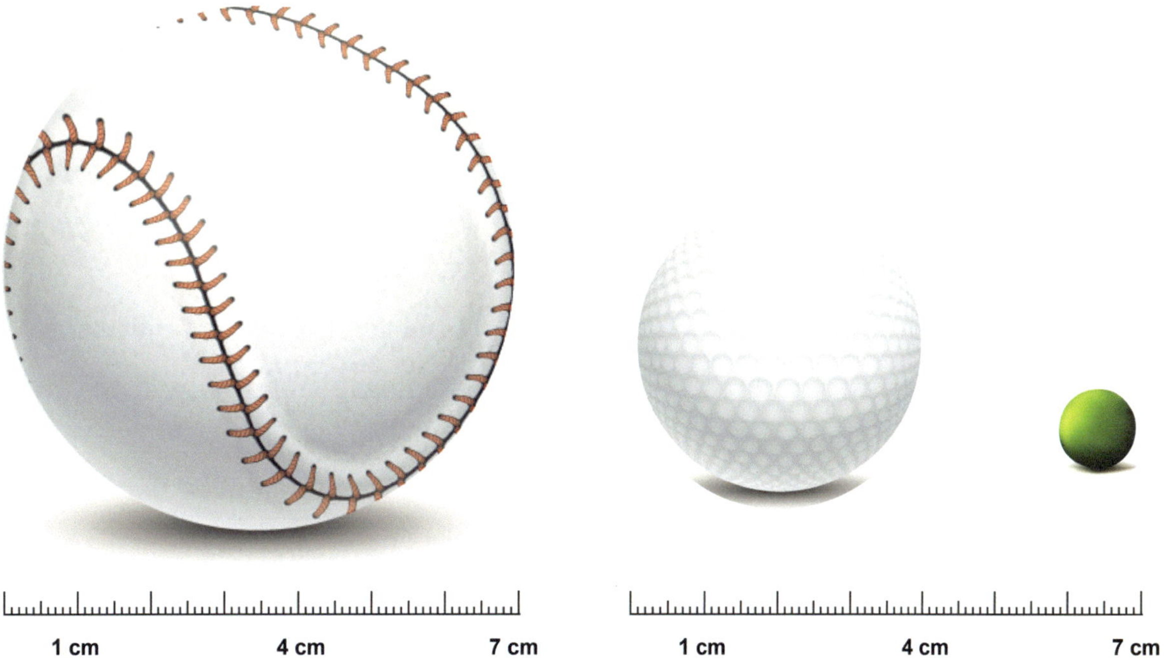

"Take things one day or even one step at a time–it might get harder before it gets better, but it will get better."

Testing and treatment

Imaging and other tests will be done to learn more about the tumor. Treatment is based on tumor size, if the tumor has spread to any nearby areas, and if the tumor might be benign (not cancer) or cancer. Tumors are usually measured in centimeters (cm). A golf ball is about 4 cm, and a large pea is about 1 cm.

- **If your tumor is less than 4 cm** and doesn't look like cancer, you'll have surgery to remove one or both adrenal glands, called an adrenalectomy. A minimally invasive surgery is preferred.
- **If your tumor is 4 cm or larger**, has grown into nearby areas, or might be cancer (adrenocortical carcinoma), you'll have an open adrenalectomy. During the procedure, your surgeon will remove the tumor, adrenal gland, and any areas where the cancer has spread, such as lymph nodes or nearby structures. For more information on adrenocortical carcinoma, see the Treatment section on page 35 in *Chapter 6, Adrenocortical carcinoma*.

Key points

- Cortisol is a hormone made and released by the adrenal glands. It helps the body use glucose (a sugar), protein, and fats. A tumor in the adrenal gland can cause hypercortisolism. Hypercortisolism occurs when your body is exposed to too much cortisol.
- When the body is exposed to hypercortisolism over a long period of time, a condition called Cushing syndrome can develop. Without treatment, Cushing syndrome can cause facial roundness, weight gain around the middle body and upper back, thinning of the arms and legs, easy bruising, and stretch marks.
- Treatment for hypercortisolism is based on tumor size, if the tumor has spread to any nearby areas, and if the tumor might be benign (not cancer) or cancer. Treatment is surgery to remove the tumor and adrenal gland. Nearby lymph nodes or other structures might be removed.

Questions to ask

- What treatment(s) do you recommend and why?
- What can I expect from treatment?
- Will I have surgery and if so, what type of surgery?
- What will be removed during surgery?
- Will I have any treatment for follow-up testing after surgery?

6

Adrenocortical carcinoma

Adrenocortical carcinoma (ACC) is cancer that forms in the outer layer of the adrenal gland called the adrenal cortex. These tumors often make and release excess hormones. Treatment aims to prevent the spread of cancer. It is usually surgery to remove the adrenal gland, tumor, or metastases.

Overview

Adrenocortical carcinoma (ACC) is cancer that forms in the cortex (outer layer) of the adrenal glands.

There are 2 types of ACC:

- **Functioning** tumors cause the adrenal gland to make excess hormones. Overproduction of cortisol and androgens is most common. Tumors can secrete more than one hormone. Most ACCs are functioning. Not all ACCs cause symptoms.
- **Nonfunctioning** tumors don't affect hormone production, but they can grow large and press on nearby organs and tissues.

In some cases, ACC has been linked to genetic conditions such as:

- Li-Fraumeni syndrome
- Lynch syndrome
- Multiple endocrine neoplasia type 1 (MEN1)
- Familial adenomatous polyposis (FAP)

Guide 3
Adrenocortical carcinoma (ACC): Systemic therapy options

Preferred therapies	• Carboplatin with etoposide (Etopophos). Doxorubicin and/or mitotane (Lysodren) might be added. • Cisplatin with etoposide. Doxorubicin and/or mitotane might be added.
Other recommended therapies	• Cabozantinib (Cabometyx) • Mitotane (Lysodren) • Pembrolizumab (Keytruda). Mitotane might be added.
Therapies used in certain cases	• Nivolumab (Opdivo) with ipilimumab (Yervoy) • Osilodrostat (Isturisa) for symptom control

Genetic counseling and testing for inherited genetic syndromes might be done if a genetic cause for an ACC is suspected.

Testing

You will have imaging scans and other tests to learn more about your cancer. Biochemical tests will be done to see if the tumor is secreting hormones such as cortisol, aldosterone, and androgen. Tumor mutation tests might also be done.

Treatment

Treatment for ACC depends on whether the tumor can be removed with surgery (resectable) or can't be removed with surgery (unresectable).

If you want and can have surgery, an open adrenalectomy is recommended. This is surgery that uses a large incision to remove the tumor and any areas where the cancer has spread, such as lymph nodes or nearby structures. After surgery, if there's a high risk that cancer might return, a clinical trial is recommended or radiation therapy to the area where the tumor was removed is possible.

If you have unresectable or metastatic disease, you may be treated with one or more of the following:

- Observation, in some cases
- Surgery (resection) to remove the main tumor and any metastases
- Radiation therapy, ablation, or arterially directed therapy to treat the main tumor or metastases
- Systemic therapy, **see Guide 3**
- Enrollment in a clinical trial

Adrenal gland

This image shows a detailed view of the outer layer (adrenal cortex) and the inner layer (medulla) of the adrenal gland. Certain hormones are produced in each zone or zona.

https://upload.wikimedia.org/wikipedia/commons/8/88/Adrenal_Gland_detail_-_English.png

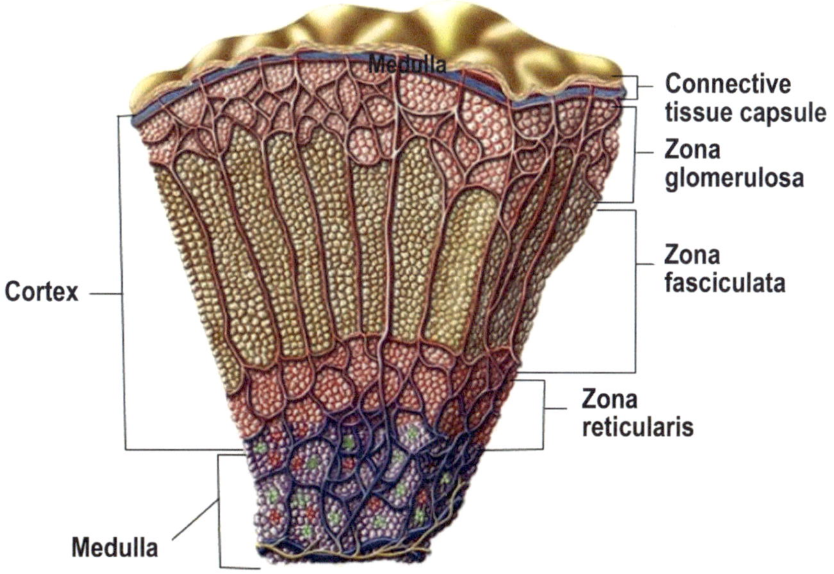

Surveillance

After treatment, you'll be monitored for signs that cancer has returned, grown, or spread. You should expect imaging tests such as CT or MRI scans every 12 weeks to 1 year. Surveillance might last 5 years or more.

Key points

- Adrenocortical carcinoma (ACC) is a cancer that forms in the cortex (outer layer) of the adrenal glands.
- Most ACCs occur randomly (not due to a genetic risk factor), but genetic testing is often offered to those with ACC.
- Primary treatment for ACC depends on whether the tumor can be removed with surgery (resectable) or can't be removed with surgery (unresectable).
- Surveillance tests are done at specific times after treatment to check if the cancer has returned.

Questions to ask

- Can the tumor be removed with surgery? Why or why not?
- What might be removed during surgery?
- If surgery isn't an option, what treatment(s) do you recommend and why?
- What are the treatment side effects?
- Is there a clinical trial available?

7 Paragaglioma and pheochromocytoma

Paraganglioma is a tumor that arises from neuroendocrine tissues found along the spine. Pheochromocytoma is a type of paraganglioma that forms in the center of the adrenal gland causing the adrenal gland to make too much adrenaline. Paragangliomas and pheochromocytomas can occur in individuals with other inherited disorders, such as von Hippel-Lindau syndrome.

Overview

This section provides an overview of paragangliomas, pheochromocytomas, and inherited conditions that might put one at increased risk for developing these tumors.

Paraganglioma

Paraganglioma (PGL) is a rare type of tumor that forms near blood vessels and nerves outside of the adrenal glands. The nerve cells affected are part of the peripheral nervous system, which is outside of the brain and spinal cord.

Paragangliomas can be found anywhere along the spine from the base of the skull to the pelvis. However, this chapter will only discuss paragangliomas found near or outside the adrenal gland. Paragangliomas can spread to other areas of the body such as lymph nodes, bones, the lung, or the liver.

"Connecting with other people with adrenal tumors—virtually and in-person—is vital to my wellbeing. This journey can feel lonely at times, and it helps so much to share thoughts and experiences with people who also struggle sometimes and understand."

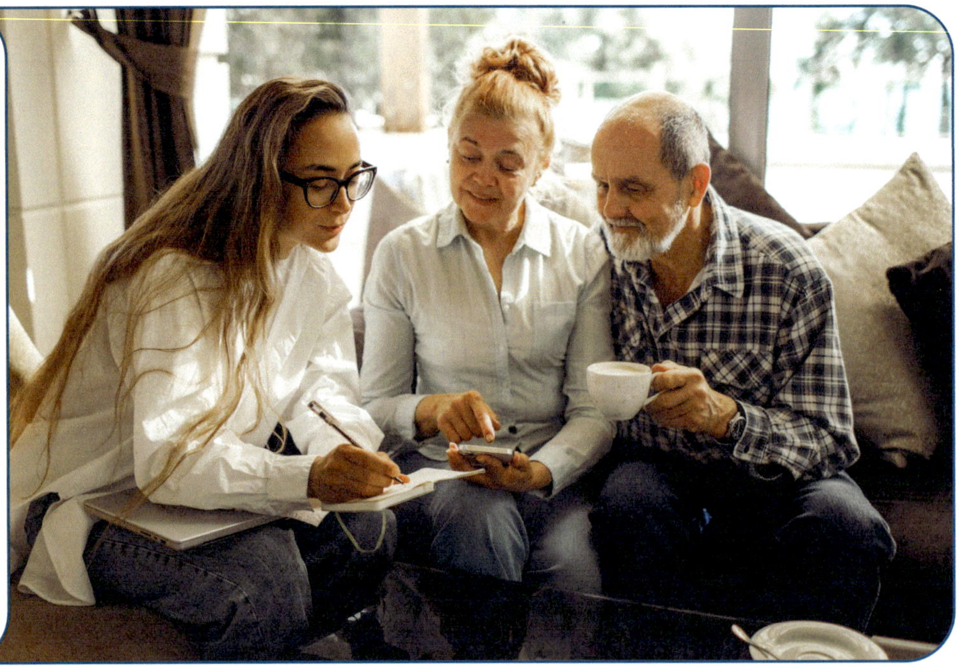

Pheochromocytoma

Pheochromocytoma (PCC) is a rare, usually benign (not cancer) tumor that develops in the center of the adrenal gland. In pheochromocytoma, the tumor grows from chromaffin cells. Chromaffin cells produce hormones including adrenaline (epinephrine) and noradrenaline (norepinephrine).

Adrenaline and noradrenaline hormones trigger your body's fight-or-flight response to act quickly to a threat. This response includes an increase in blood pressure and a rapid heartbeat. Pheochromocytoma causes these hormones to be released, even when you are not in a threatening situation.

A pheochromocytoma (or "pheo" for short) can cause high blood pressure, pounding headaches, irregular heartbeat, flushing of the face, sweating, nausea, and vomiting.

Inherited conditions

Some rare hereditary conditions can increase the risk for paraganglioma and pheochromocytoma.

These inherited conditions include:

- Hereditary pheochromocytoma/ paraganglioma (PCC/PGL) syndrome
- Multiple endocrine neoplasia type 2 (MEN2)
- Neurofibromatosis type 1 (NF1)
- Von Hippel-Lindau (VHL) syndrome

Testing

Tests such as imaging scans, blood, urine, and tumor mutation tests will be used to diagnose a paraganglioma or pheochromocytoma and plan treatment. Genetic counseling and testing for inherited genetic syndromes might be done if a genetic cause is suspected. Most people with PGL or PCC are offered genetic testing.

Treatment

Before starting treatment, you'll likely be prescribed alpha blockers to lower your blood pressure. Types of alpha blockers include alpha 1 selective receptor blockers such as terazosin, doxazosin, and prazosin, and non-selective receptor blockers such as phenoxybenzamine. You'll also be asked to eat a high salt diet and drink a lot of fluids for a few days before procedures such as surgery.

One or more of the following medicines might be added to the alpha blockers:

- Dihydropyridine calcium channel blocker
- Beta blocker
- Metyrosine

Treatment is based on if the tumor can be removed with surgery (resectable) or can't be removed with surgery (unresectable), if the tumor is making and releasing hormones, and if tumors have spread to other areas of the body (metastases) such as the lymph nodes, bones, the lung, or the liver. Pheochromocytomas rarely spread.

Treatment options are described next.

- **For a resectable tumor**, minimally invasive surgery is recommended whenever possible.
- **For an unresectable tumor or distant metastases** not causing symptoms (asymptomatic) or slow growing, your condition will be monitored for any changes. This is called observation.
- **For an unresectable tumor** that's secreting hormones, you'll continue taking the alpha blocker, and options include a clinical trial, radiation therapy, and possible surgery to reduce the tumor size, or systemic therapy.
- **For distant metastases** that are secreting hormones, you'll continue taking the alpha blocker, and options include a clinical trial, surgery to reduce the tumor size, systemic therapy, or radiation therapy to treat metastases or metastases causing symptoms.

Systemic therapy options can be found in **Guide 4.**

Guide 4 Systemic therapy options
Clinical trial
Belzutifan (Welireg)
Cabozantinib (Cabometyx)
High-specific-activity (HSA) iobenguane I-131 or other 131I-MIBG
Selpercatinib (Retevmo)
Sunitinib (Sutent)
Cyclophosphamide, vincristine, and dacarbazine (CVD) or temozolomide (Temodar)
PRRT with lutetium Lu 177 dotatate (Lutathera) if tumor is SSTR-positive
SSAs (octreotide LAR or lanreotide) if tumor is SSTR-positive

Surveillance

Surveillance tests are done at specific times after treatment to check on any changes in your condition. You can expect to have blood and urine tests and to have your blood pressure monitored regularly. Imaging tests are possible, with a CT or MRI being most common. Other imaging tests are possible.

Key points

- Paraganglioma (PGL) is a rare type of tumor that forms near blood vessels and nerves outside of the adrenal gland.
- Pheochromocytoma (PCC) is a rare, usually benign tumor that develops in the center of the adrenal gland causing the adrenal gland to make too much adrenaline.
- You may be at risk for PGL or PCC if you have a rare inherited condition. Tumors associated with these disorders are more likely to be cancer. Most people with PGL or PCC are offered genetic testing.
- You will have blood, urine, and imaging tests to diagnose a PGL or PCC.
- Some people who have PGL or PCC will develop symptoms, while others will not. The most common symptom is hypertension (high blood pressure).
- Before treatment, you will likely be prescribed medicine (alpha blockers) to lower your blood pressure. You'll also be asked to eat a high salt diet and drink a lot of fluids for a few days before procedures such as surgery.
- Surveillance tests are done at specific times after treatment to check if the cancer has returned.

Questions to ask

- What type of tumor do I have?
- Is the tumor producing any hormones?
- What are my treatment options?
- What treatment(s) do you recommend and why?
- What are the treatment side effects?

We want your feedback!

Our goal is to provide helpful and easy-to-understand information on cancer. Take our survey to let us know what we got right and what we could do better. NCCN.org/patients/feedback

8
Other resources

Want to learn more? Here's how you can get additional help.

What else to know

This book helps you know your options so you can make informed decisions and improve your cancer care. But it's not the only resource that you have.

Ask for as much information and help as you need. Many people are interested in learning more about:

- Finding an oncologist or doctor who's an expert in adrenal tumors
- Making treatment decisions
- The details of treatment and its side effects
- Getting financial help
- Coping with other health challenges

What else to do

Your health care center can help you with next steps. It often has on-site resources to help meet your needs and find answers to your questions. Health care centers can also inform you of resources in your community.

In addition to help from your providers, the resources listed in the next section provide support for many people like yourself.

Where to get help

Look through the list below and visit the provided websites to learn more about these organizations.

Bone Marrow & Cancer Foundation
bonemarrow.org

CancerCare
cancercare.org

Imerman Angels
Imermanangels.org

MedlinePlus
medlineplus.gov

National Cancer Institute (NCI)
cancer.gov

Neuroendocrine Cancer Awareness Network
netcancerawareness.org

Neuroendocrine Tumor Research Foundation
netrf.org

The Healing NET Foundation
thehealingnet.org

Triage Cancer
triagecancer.org

Questions to ask

- Who can I talk to about help with housing, food, and other basic needs?
- What help is available for transportation, childcare, and home care?
- What other services are available to me and my caregivers?
- How can I connect with others and build a support system?
- Who can I talk to if I don't feel safe at home, at work, or in my neighborhood?

Finding a clinical trial

In the United States

NCCN Cancer Centers
NCCN.org/cancercenters

The National Cancer Institute (NCI)
cancer.gov/about-cancer/treatment/clinical-trials/search

Worldwide

The U.S. National Library of Medicine (NLM)
clinicaltrials.gov/

Need help finding a clinical trial?

NCI's Cancer Information Service (CIS)
1.800.4.CANCER (1.800.422.6237)
cancer.gov/contact

Words to know

adrenal cortex
The outer layer of the adrenal gland that makes androgen and corticosteroid hormones.

adrenalectomy
Surgery to remove one or both adrenal glands.

adrenal gland
A small organ on top of each kidney that makes hormones.

adrenocortical carcinoma (ACC)
A rare type of cancer that forms in the adrenal cortex (outer layer) of the adrenal glands.

biochemical test
A test to measure the level of chemicals in the body.

biomarker
A substance found in body tissue or fluid that may be a sign of cancer.

biopsy
A procedure that removes fluid or tissue samples to be tested for disease.

carcinoma
A cancer of cells that line the inner or outer surfaces of the body.

chemotherapy
Drugs that kill cancer cells by damaging or disrupting the making of the genetic code.

clinical trial
A type of research that assesses health tests or treatments.

computed tomography (CT)
A test that uses x-rays from many angles to make pictures of the inside of the body.

Conn syndrome
A condition that occurs due to too much aldosterone being produced by the adrenal glands. Also called primary aldosteronism or hyperaldosteronism.

contrast
A substance put into your body to make clearer pictures during imaging tests.

cortisol
A hormone that controls blood sugar, metabolism, and other functions in the body.

Cushing syndrome
A condition caused by the release of excess cortisol in the body over a long period of time.

gene
Coded instructions in cells for making new cells and controlling how cells behave.

hereditary
Passed down from birth parent to child through coded information in cells.

hormone
A chemical in the body that triggers a response from cells or organs.

hypercortisolism
A condition caused by the release of excess cortisol in the body.

hypertension
A condition in which the force of the blood against the artery walls is too high. Also referred to as high blood pressure.

imaging
A test that makes pictures (images) of the insides of the body.

immunotherapy
A treatment with drugs that help the body find and destroy cancer cells.

lymph node
A small, bean-shaped disease-fighting structure.

magnetic resonance imaging (MRI)
A test that uses radio waves and powerful magnets to make pictures of the insides of the body.

metastasis
The spread of cancer cells from the first (primary) tumor to a new site.

mutation
An abnormal change in cells.

observation
A period of testing for changes in cancer status while not receiving treatment.

palliative care
Health care that includes symptom relief but not cancer treatment. Also sometimes called supportive care.

paraganglioma (PGL)
A tumor that arises from neuroendocrine tissues found along the spine.

pheochromocytoma (PCC)
A tumor that forms in the center of the adrenal gland that causes it to make too much adrenaline.

positron emission tomography (PET)
A test that uses radioactive material to see the shape and function of body parts.

primary aldosteronism
A condition that occurs due to too much aldosterone being produced by the adrenal glands. Also called Conn syndrome or hyperaldosteronism.

primary treatment
The main treatment used to rid the body of cancer.

primary tumor
The first mass of cancer cells.

progression
The growth or spread of cancer after being tested or treated.

radiation therapy (RT)
A treatment that uses high-energy rays or related approaches to kill cancer cells.

radiopharmaceutical
A drug that carries a certain amount of radioactive material.

somatostatin
A hormone that attaches to receptors and controls the endocrine system and nervous system.

somatostatin analogs (SSAs)
A treatment used to slow down or stop tumor hormone production.

somatostatin receptor (SSTR)
Found on some types of tumors and causes the tumor to release extra hormones.

supportive care
Health care that includes symptom relief but not cancer treatment. Also called palliative care.

surgery
An operation to remove or repair a part of the body.

surgical margin
The normal-looking tissue around the edge of a tumor that is removed during surgery.

targeted therapy
A drug treatment that impedes the growth process specific to cancer cells.

NCCN Contributors

This patient guide is based on the NCCN Clinical Practice Guidelines in Oncology (NCCN Guidelines®) for Neuroendocrine and Adrenal Tumors Version 2.2025. It was adapted, reviewed, and published with help from the following people:

Dorothy A. Shead, MS
Senior Director
Patient Information Operations

Tanya Fischer, MEd, MSLIS
Senior Medical Writer

Lisa Diehl
Production Layout Artist

The NCCN Clinical Practice Guidelines in Oncology (NCCN Guidelines®) for Neuroendocrine and Adrenal Tumors Version 2.2025 were developed by the following NCCN Panel Members:

*Emily Bergsland, MD/Chair
UCSF Helen Diller Family Comprehensive Cancer Center

J. Bart Rose, MD/Vice Chair
O'Neal Comprehensive Cancer Center at UAB

Al B. Benson III, MD
Robert H. Lurie Comprehensive Cancer Center of Northwestern University

Zachary Berman, MD
UC San Diego Moores Cancer Center

Lawrence S. Blaszkowsky, MD
Dana-Farber/Brigham and Women's Cancer Center | Mass General Cancer Center

*Pamela Brock, MS
The Ohio State University Comprehensive Cancer Center - James Cancer Hospital and Solove Research Institute

Jennifer Chan, MD
Dana-Farber/Brigham and Women's Cancer Center | Mass General Cancer Center

Deyali Chatterjee, MD
The University of Texas MD Anderson Cancer Center

*Paxton V. Dickson, MD
The University of Tennessee Health Science Center

Abbey Fingeret, MD, MHPTT
Fred & Pamela Buffett Cancer Center

Apar Kishor P. Ganti, MD
Fred & Pamela Buffett Cancer Center

*Phillip Ge, MD
The University of Texas MD Anderson Cancer Center

Mark Girgis, MD
UCLA Jonsson Comprehensive Cancer Center

Thorvardur R. Halfdanarson, MD
Mayo Clinic Comprehensive Cancer Center

Christopher L. Hallemeier, MD
Mayo Clinic Comprehensive Cancer Center

Jin He, MD, PhD
Johns Hopkins Kimmel Cancer Center

Rong Hu, MD
University of Wisconsin Carbone Cancer Center

Shruti Jolly, MD, MBA
University of Michigan Rogel Cancer Center

Fouad Kandeel, MD, PhD
City of Hope National Medical Center

Syed M. Kazmi, MD
UT Southwestern Simmons Comprehensive Cancer Center

Xavier Keutgen, MD
The UChicago Medicine Comprehensive Cancer Center

Sajid A. Khan, MD
Yale Cancer Center/ Smilow Cancer Hospital

Christopher Lieu, MD
University of Colorado Cancer Center

Amr Mohamed, MD
Case Comprehensive Cancer Center/ University Hospitals Seidman Cancer Center and Cleveland Clinic Taussig Cancer Institute

Shaffer Mok, MD
Moffitt Cancer Center

Nitya Raj, MD
Memorial Sloan Kettering Cancer Center

Fatma Sen, MD, MSc
UC Davis Comprehensive Cancer Center

Shagufta Shaheen, MD
Stanford Cancer Institute

Heloisa P. Soares, MD, PhD
Huntsman Cancer Institute at the University of Utah

Michael C. Soulen, MD
Abramson Cancer Center at the University of Pennsylvania

Zachary Stiles, DO, MS
Roswell Park Comprehensive Cancer Center

Jonathan R. Strosberg, MD
Moffitt Cancer Center

Craig R. Sussman, MD
Vanderbilt-Ingram Cancer Center

Nikolaos A. Trikalinos, MD
Siteman Cancer Center at Barnes-Jewish Hospital and Washington University School of Medicine

Namrata Vijayvergia, MD
Fox Chase Cancer Center

Terence Wong, MD, PhD
Duke Cancer Institute

Anthony Yang, MD, MS, FACS
Indiana University Melvin and Bren Simon Comprehensive Cancer Center

David B. Zhen, MD
Fred Hutchinson Cancer Center

NCCN

Cindy Hochstetler, PhD
Oncology Scientist/Senior Medical Writer

Beth McCullough, RN, BS
Guidelines Coordinator

* Reviewed this patient guide. For disclosures, visit NCCN.org/disclosures.

NCCN Cancer Centers

Abramson Cancer Center
at the University of Pennsylvania
Philadelphia, Pennsylvania
800.789.7366 • pennmedicine.org/cancer

Case Comprehensive Cancer Center/
University Hospitals Seidman Cancer Center and
Cleveland Clinic Taussig Cancer Institute
Cleveland, Ohio
UH Seidman Cancer Center
800.641.2422 • uhhospitals.org/services/cancer-services
CC Taussig Cancer Institute
866.223.8100 • my.clevelandclinic.org/departments/cancer
Case CCC
216.844.8797 • case.edu/cancer

City of Hope National Medical Center
Duarte, California
800.826.4673 • cityofhope.org

Dana-Farber/Brigham and Women's Cancer Center |
Mass General Cancer Center
Boston, Massachusetts
877.442.3324 • youhaveus.org
617.726.5130 • massgeneral.org/cancer-center

Duke Cancer Institute
Durham, North Carolina
888.275.3853 • dukecancerinstitute.org

Fox Chase Cancer Center
Philadelphia, Pennsylvania
888.369.2427 • foxchase.org

Fred & Pamela Buffett Cancer Center
Omaha, Nebraska
402.559.5600 • unmc.edu/cancercenter

Fred Hutchinson Cancer Center
Seattle, Washington
206.667.5000 • fredhutch.org

Huntsman Cancer Institute at the University of Utah
Salt Lake City, Utah
800.824.2073 • healthcare.utah.edu/huntsmancancerinstitute

Indiana University Melvin and Bren Simon
Comprehensive Cancer Center
Indianapolis, Indiana
888.600.4822 • www.cancer.iu.edu

Johns Hopkins Kimmel Cancer Center
Baltimore, Maryland
410.955.8964
www.hopkinskimmelcancercenter.org

Mayo Clinic Comprehensive Cancer Center
Phoenix/Scottsdale, Arizona
Jacksonville, Florida
Rochester, Minnesota
480.301.8000 • Arizona
904.953.0853 • Florida
507.538.3270 • Minnesota
mayoclinic.org/cancercenter

Memorial Sloan Kettering Cancer Center
New York, New York
800.525.2225 • mskcc.org

Moffitt Cancer Center
Tampa, Florida
888.663.3488 • moffitt.org

O'Neal Comprehensive Cancer Center at UAB
Birmingham, Alabama
800.822.0933 • uab.edu/onealcancercenter

Robert H. Lurie Comprehensive Cancer Center
of Northwestern University
Chicago, Illinois
866.587.4322 • cancer.northwestern.edu

Roswell Park Comprehensive Cancer Center
Buffalo, New York
877.275.7724 • roswellpark.org

Siteman Cancer Center at Barnes-Jewish Hospital
and Washington University School of Medicine
St. Louis, Missouri
800.600.3606 • siteman.wustl.edu

St. Jude Children's Research Hospital/
The University of Tennessee Health Science Center
Memphis, Tennessee
866.278.5833 • stjude.org
901.448.5500 • uthsc.edu

Stanford Cancer Institute
Stanford, California
877.668.7535 • cancer.stanford.edu

The Ohio State University Comprehensive Cancer Center -
James Cancer Hospital and Solove Research Institute
Columbus, Ohio
800.293.5066 • cancer.osu.edu

The UChicago Medicine Comprehensive Cancer Center
Chicago, Illinois
773.702.1000 • uchicagomedicine.org/cancer

The University of Texas MD Anderson Cancer Center
Houston, Texas
844.269.5922 • mdanderson.org

UC Davis Comprehensive Cancer Center
Sacramento, California
916.734.5959 • 800.770.9261
health.ucdavis.edu/cancer

UC San Diego Moores Cancer Center
La Jolla, California
858.822.6100 • cancer.ucsd.edu

UCLA Jonsson Comprehensive Cancer Center
Los Angeles, California
310.825.5268 • uclahealth.org/cancer

UCSF Helen Diller Family
Comprehensive Cancer Center
San Francisco, California
800.689.8273 • cancer.ucsf.edu

University of Colorado Cancer Center
Aurora, Colorado
720.848.0300 • coloradocancercenter.org

University of Michigan Rogel Cancer Center
Ann Arbor, Michigan
800.865.1125 • rogelcancercenter.org

University of Wisconsin Carbone Cancer Center
Madison, Wisconsin
608.265.1700 • uwhealth.org/cancer

UT Southwestern Simmons
Comprehensive Cancer Center
Dallas, Texas
214.648.3111 • utsouthwestern.edu/simmons

Vanderbilt-Ingram Cancer Center
Nashville, Tennessee
877.936.8422 • vicc.org

Yale Cancer Center/Smilow Cancer Hospital
New Haven, Connecticut
855.4.SMILOW • yalecancercenter.org

share with us.

Take our survey and help make the NCCN Guidelines for Patients better for everyone!

NCCN.org/patients/comments

Notes

Index

Made in the USA
Monee, IL
05 November 2026

67382563R00033